Your First Makeup

Experience: Makeup Basics

and Tips for Young Girls

Monica C. Falco

Table of Contents

While I was the 7th grade, I became interested in makeup. I was rather curious about it, and so I decided that I wanted to start buying some to play around with. To my surprise, my best friend decided to buy me a big bag of makeup for my birthday! I was ever so excited, and I dove right into application. I tried different techniques and colors on for hours on end until my face was sore. Included in the big bag were a variety of different eye shadow colors, a couple lip glosses, mascara, an eyelash curler, some blush, and a charcoal colored eyeliner pencil. I decided to put the metallic light blue eye shadow over my eyelids, I put the eyeliner on my bottom eye lid, and I put on the mascara lightly and curled my eyelashes. I remember feeling so mature and powerful when I looked at myself in the mirror.

After experimenting with this makeup for a few days, I then started to wear makeup to school occasionally. I found a technique that I liked, so I decided, "This is how I'm going to wear it." It was very bright makeup that I chose. My eyelids were always bright blue, and my lips were always light pink and full of shiny gloss.

When you're in elementary school or younger, you probably received makeup as a gift for Christmas from your parents or for your birthday. The makeup was probably bright, Barbie-doll like makeup. The lip gloss was fire-truck red, the eye shadow was bright pink, and the blush was purple and full of glitter. You knew that Barbie was beautiful and you loved her makeup! Five or six years later, perhaps you are cleaning out your room getting rid of toys that you have grown too old for. You might come across a Barbie doll and notice her magenta pink lips. You might ask yourself why her lips are magenta pink and her eye shadow bright purple. From what you have observed, girls don't wear makeup that looks like Barbie's! And the truth be told, they really don't!

Many girls in the junior high age range start becoming interested in makeup and start to wonder how to wear it, and what to wear. They feel lost, though- because they do not know how to apply makeup correctly. They don't know what colors to wear, what kind to buy, or how much to wear. Let alone, they don't know what components go where on the face. Since Barbie served as a role model for many young girls, girls might not understand that makeup is not meant to be bright and flashy, but rather feature enhancing and natural looking. However, there are big problems us young girls go through when starting out with makeup. We usually start off wearing too much, wearing the wrong colors, or applying it all wrong! In this book, you will learn all of the basics of makeup needed to be a successful learner on the subject of makeup. You will learn what colors look best on your skin and features, and you will learn how to apply makeup correctly in the form of eye shadow, mascara, foundations, blush, and more.

Also, you must start your makeup routine with clean skin and at bedtime proper removal to keep your skin healthy, which you will also learn. I have even included an extra chapter on the "5 common mistakes with makeup". If you're at the age where you are getting interested in makeup and are anxious to learn about proper application, then this book is a must for you!

Chapter One: What is makeup?

What do you think makeup is? Many people have different definitions of what it is. Some say it's a form of art, some say it's unnatural, some say it's a mask. But I say that's it's a natural feature enhancing tool, because it is! Makeup is the simple art of enhancing one's features. It is not, however, meant to completely alter the way you look. If it's completely altering the way you naturally look, it is probably an indicator that you're wearing too much makeup. As stated above, makeup is a tool used to pull attention to the features on the face. These features include the eyes, the cheekbones, the lips, the eyelashes, eyebrows, the nose, and the overall skin of a girl's face. Bringing attention to the features can come in the form of colors, amounts, textures, and depth.

Makeup can also be used for different purposes in different ways. The bright and attention-getter looking makeup for a ballet play uses a different style of makeup versus the makeup attire for everyday school. The reason there are so many makeup choices at the stores are for this very reason. If you go to Wal-Mart and look at their makeup selection, there are nearly 5 isles full of different makeup brands, providing a huge variety of colors for every makeup component. Makeup is truly an art form and practice in itself, and most girls find the makeup adventure very exciting and full of fun, as I'm

sure you will as well. Learning how to properly

apply makeup is going to take some practice,

too. Once you get down the proper techniques,

all of your friends and peers will be asking you

how you learned to makeup so well.

Chapter 2: Intro to Makeup components and their roles

In this chapter, I will outline the uses of the

various makeup components. In chapter 5, I will

discuss how to properly apply all the

components. There are many different

components and kinds of makeup that are

available for purchase and use. These include

eye shadow, foundation, blush, eyeliner,

mascara, and lip wear. We are going to go down the list, starting with eye shadow.

Eye shadow is used to bring out the color of the eyes, or it can be used to serve as soft looking eyeliner. There are a few different eye shadow placement techniques. Some people put eye shadow over their entire eyelid, some put it only in the corner of the eyes (closest to the nose), some put it only in the outer corner of the eyes, and some put it all over their eyelid along with their brow bone (the area below the eyebrow). These different placement techniques serve different purposes in enhancing the eyes.

Eyeliner, another eye tool, is used to intensify and define your eyes. Typically, eyeliner is placed underneath the eye, outlining the lower eyelid. If a girl wants extra definition and intensity, she can line up eyeliner against her top eyelid, too, right over top of the eyelash line. For makeup beginners, eyeliner is generally preferred for only the lower lid, as it creates the look of natural, minimal makeup.

Mascara is another eye-enhancing tool. Mascara goes on the tip of your eyelashes. It brightens the color of the eyes, bringing attention to your eye color. It also lengthens your eyelashes dramatically or slightly, depending on which brand/which kind you apply.

Now were going to discuss the various facial components of makeup. Blush is a coloring tool used to brighten up your cheeks. It's generally used to bring attention to your cheekbones and your eyes. Blush is a little bit difficult to learn to use for beginners, so it's important that you learn how to properly apply it, as I will discuss in chapter 5. When I was in middle school, I made the mistake of thinking blush went all over my face. One day a girl pointed it out, as I was quite embarrassed! In that moment I had wished I had had a proper learning about makeup in my younger days.

Foundation is another facial makeup component. Foundation is the base for all of your makeup. There are many different colors and forms of foundation including liquid, pressed powder, liquid powder, and loose powder. It's important to learn how to use foundation correctly, as well as blush. These two go hand and hand together and must blend so that they complement each other. You will need to find a shade that matches your skin tone and one that blends with your skin and looks natural.

Foundation can be tricky to apply, so it's very important to learn proper technique! Foundation pulls together all of your makeup components, which is why you always want to put it on before anything else. Right after you wash your face, you want to put on your foundation. Important tip: blush goes on lastly! When you're wearing blush and foundation together, your complexion is meant to look soft, blended, natural, and full of glow.

Lip wear can come in the form of lip gloss or lip stick. It gives away its role in its name. Many lip wear products are made with moisturizer for your lips, while others are not. If you typically suffer from chap lips, you'll want to pick out lip glosses with moisturizer in them. Again, there are many different brands and colors of lip wear out there. When you're picking it out, keep in mind whether or not you need one with or without moisturizing properties. In my experience, I have bought some lip glosses that completely dry my lips out because my lips are naturally chapped. So a word of warning, definitely watch out for that!

Chapter 3: Preparing Skin for Makeup & Removal

Before you apply any kind of makeup, it's extremely important that you have a clean, moisturized face. If your face is not moisturized and clean, your makeup will look dull, chalky, and flaky- and some of it might easily rub off. Not only that, but your pores will become super clogged up with dirt, oil and makeup if you don't clean and moisturize your skin before and after makeup application, eventually leading to annoying breakouts on your face. Your skin tone will also most likely be uneven looking. Keeping your face moisturized on a daily basis is important not only in maintaining healthy skin, but also for smooth application of any makeup. Just as important, your face must be clean! Before you put on your makeup in the morning, make sure to clean your face with cold water/lukewarm water and soap. Don't use hot water because it will quickly dry out your skin. Lather cold/lukewarm water on your face with soap, and let it sit for about two minutes. Then, rinse your face carefully, avoiding eye contact with the soapy water. After you're finished rinsing your face, dry it off with a towel completely. After your face is clean, put a light layer of preferably unscented lotion onto your face. This will ensure that your makeup goes on smooth and you'll also avoid makeup lines when your skin is soft and hydrated. After this cleansing and hydrating process, you'll have a clean face to apply makeup to, assuring the smoothest, best application. This process will eventually become habit for you, and it is not very time consuming for its amazing benefits. It's very practical, and a great solution to preventing acne.

At night time, to remove your makeup, follow these instructions. I live by these instructions, and have used these tips for years and years! I made the mistake of buying makeup removing pads, which most girls do. After a while I found that these makeup removing pads were too expensive and so I tried other things to try to get my makeup off. And I sure did find one. It's a cheaper, more natural alternative, and doesn't get your face all messy and smeary, unlike makeup removing pads. To remove your eye makeup in a clean manner, (eyeliner, mascara, eye shadow) take a cotton ball and dip it into a jar of Vaseline. Vaseline serves as a moisturizer, and also takes eye makeup off easily in a clear, clean way- much more than the mainstream makeup removing pads. Once you have your dipped cotton ball in Vaseline, gently wipe it back and forth horizontally over your eyes with your eyes closed, of course. After rubbing your eyes for 30 seconds or so, the makeup should be gone off your eyes, and onto the cotton ball. You will notice that your skin around your eyes is slippery, covered in Vaseline. (Tip: I leave Vaseline on my eyelashes only when I sleep, because it makes them slightly grow.) After you've taken your eye makeup off, you'll want to rinse your face now, with soap and water to take off the foundation or blush you were wearing. Tip: you never, ever want to go to bed with any form of makeup on your face! If you sleep in mascara, your eyelashes will start to thin out, and eventually start falling out. It's extremely important to take off all eye makeup for this reason. You also never want to go to bed with any kind of foundation or blush on! If you do, this will immensely clog your pores and create acne the next morning. This is why you must wash your face with soap and water before you go to bed. If your face is feeling dry, apply some lotion to lock in moisture. And there you have it: the proper way to clean your face before and after makeup application.

Chapter 4: Finding your shades and colors

Finding your matching foundation shade can be a challenge at first. When you go to a store that sells makeup, you might be overwhelmed by all the brand choices and colors and types of makeup. Finding your foundation and blush shade is tricky because you want one to look the most natural on you. The variety of foundation types is nearly endless. Foundation comes in the form of liquid, pressed liquid powder, loose powder, and pressed powder. Since you're a makeup beginner, I recommend pressed powder. Pressed powder is the easiest of them all to apply, and it is the least time-consuming to apply. Until you get down the advanced techniques of foundation such as liquid, I would stick with pressed powder for the time being. I typically recommend liquid based foundations for girls that are older- at least in high school. Liquid foundation is more difficult to apply and blend on your face. Now to find your shade! If you pick a shade that's too dark for you, it will look very obvious and people will notice how your face doesn't match the rest of your body. If your shade is too light, well, it won't match your body either. You want to look natural! Since foundation is used to enhance the skin of the face, you must find the closest matching shade to your skin color. A rule of thumb for finding your shade: Always pick one shade darker than what matches your body skin in the sample color. The reason for this is because your face is naturally a tint darker than your body, since your face is the one body part that's always exposed to the sun- whether the spring, summer, or even winter. Your face always remains a tint darker than your body.

Next, I will explain the different blush colors and their purposes. First off, your blush must blend in with your foundation smoothly. You don't want two complete different colors that won't blend well. However, it's important to pick out a blush that is darker than your natural skin. Most young girls go with a pinkish colored blush. A pink blush brings out the cheeks in a rosy youthful manner.

Me personally, I go with the super natural look, and wear a light bronze blush. This color blush blends well with my foundation, and provides a super natural look. Blushes can range from red to pink to brown to a slight orange. If you want a natural look, go with the browns or super light pinks. If you want to bring your cheekbones out more, go with a darker pink or red shade of blush.

Next, we will discuss eye shadow. Eye shadows are fun to experiment with. For minimal and newbie purposes, you will want to pick out an eye shadow or two that's one solid color. If you like bright colors, try a blue, brown, or orange shade. If you want to look more natural, try a light brown, beige, light orange, white, or tan shade. Try avoiding super, intense neon looking colors-as these shades will most likely wash your face out. Tip: If you have blue eyes, brown and oranges are the colors that will make your eye color pop more than any other colors. The reasoning for this is because brown and blue are complimentary colors on the color wheel. This same rule goes with brown eyes. If you have brown eyes, blue and green eye shadows will pop your brown eyes out the most. If you have green eyes, your eyes will look lovely in lavender and light pink shadows. The girls with hazel eyes can use the same guidelines as the blue eyes or go with a neutral color. Neutral eye shadow colors of course always look good with any eye color. You can never go wrong with a neutral eye shadow.

Eyeliner is pretty easy to choose when purchasing. It comes in the form of liquid, crayon-like, and pencil. For starters, I recommend the pencil kind. It's the cheapest form of eyeliner and will last a while. If you buy pencil eyeliner, you must buy an eyeliner sharpener too. They are low in cost and needed if you're using an eyeliner pencil. Eyeliner comes in many different colors. Of these colors, the most popular ones are charcoal (gray), black, and brown. If you want a soft black look, go with the charcoal. If you want an intense look, choose the black. If you want a more natural look, go with brown. You can of course experiment with these colors to see which one you like best.

Mascara comes in the form of dark blue, black and brown. Black mascara is the most common color used. Black mascara will darken your lashes greatly. Blue mascara will add a blue tint and shine to your eyelashes, and brown will softly highlight your lashes.

Chapter 5: Applying Makeup

To apply foundation, make sure you have prepared your skin the cleansing and moisturizing process, as explained in Chapter 3. I am going to explain how to apply pressed powder foundation, as I recommended it as the beginner choice for starting foundation. Once you find your shade, you want to open your powder, and take out the brush pad included in the container. You'll want to use the fluffy side of the pad for application, not the cotton flat side. Dip a small edge of the pad into the pressed powder and start dabbing anywhere on your face with it. I personally find it easier to apply foundation to the outside of the cheeks, chin, jawbone and forehead before anywhere else, because that gives you an outline of where to fill in the rest. Tip: Do not dip the entire face pad into the powder, because it wastes powder and gives you less control over foundation placement. Make sure to apply on your nose, and also your eyelids. The reason you want to apply to your eyelids is because it serves as a base for your eye shadow. This base will keep your eye shadow on longer and keeps it smoother looking, not allowing your eye shadow to smear and develop crease lines from your eyelids. While you're putting foundation on above your eyes, close them, as you won't want to get makeup in them. You might have to dip a couple times until you have your entire face lightly covered.

After your face is full of pretty foundation, you can move on to the blush process. Whatever shade of blush you picked out, dip the brush in the powder all the way, and give yourself a big smile in the mirror! While smiling, apply the brush in a circular motion onto the apples on your cheeks. Your apples are your cheekbones that are visible when you smile. Keep in mind to not use too much blush, because you want it to blend in with your foundation. Tip: If you want to bring your cheekbones out even more, brush the brush along your temple lightly onto the apples of your cheeks.

After your blush is well blended with your foundation, you can move onto your eyes! Tip: *always* apply your eye shadow first, before any other eye makeup. When you have your color picked out, swipe a light layer over your entire eyelid. By this, I mean only apply it below the crease of your eyelid. If it gets above the crease, it will look messy and excessive. This is very important! Once your eye shadow is applied, you can apply your bottom eyelid with eyeliner. Tip: To ensure proper application, try to line the eyeliner as close to your eyeball as you can. This does not mean open up your eyelids. It means go as close as you can to your eye! (Without poking your eyes, of course.) The line should be super thin, too. If your eyeliner is too thick, it will make your eyes appear small and dull without definition.

After you have on your eye shadow and eyeliner, it's time for mascara! Mascara is one of the trickiest to apply. People often make mistakes while applying mascara. A very important tip: only apply mascara to the tips of the eyelashes. If you apply it to the entire width of eyelashes, it will weigh them down and cause them to look shorter than they really are. When you apply to just the tips, it will lengthen your lashes dramatically and your lashes will not be clumpy. You do not want to overuse mascara. The more you pile on your lashes, the more your lashes will clump together. Clumpy isn't good! Your lashes will look much more beautiful and clean if you apply a light layer of mascara. Light mascara applied to the tips of your lashes will make them look very long and natural.

There you have it: The proper way to apply the basic makeup components. Along your journey of makeup, you will quickly learn your own little tips and tricks, and what works best for you. Makeup is a big experiment stage in itself and has a learning curve to it. But now that you know the basics, start with those!

Chapter 6: Five Most Common Mistakes with Makeup

1). Too much foundation! I often see young girls that are starting to wear makeup pile it on way too much! The key to foundation and blush is minimum wear and maximum blending. If you have on too much foundation, it will look chalky and pasty. Your face will feel heavy and your pores will feel clogged up. Too much foundation and blush will overload and clog your skin, so take it easy on the application. Acne can be prevented greatly by the skin and moisturizing process, and by applying the right amount of foundation.

2) Too much Mascara! As I stated in a previous chapter, an over application of mascara is always a negative. The more you apply on your lashes, the shorter and clumpier your lashes will look. Apply mascara one time to the tips of your eyelashes, and no more! You can surely over line your lashes a couple times, but do this in the same time period. Never apply more than one coat of mascara once the first coat is dry. This will create lots of clumps and shorten them. It will

also make your mascara more difficult to take off.

3) Wearing the wrong shade of foundation. If your foundation is too dark, you will look uneven, unblended, and unnatural. I cannot emphasize the importance of picking out the correct foundation shade. On the other hand, if your foundation is too light, you won't look natural and blended, either. This is a major common mistake in makeup wear. I see it in all ages- young, middle aged, and even the elderly. The proper shade will make you look natural and beautiful, as it will compliment your skin tone. It will make all of the difference in your entire complexion.

4) Too much eye shadow. When a girl is wearing too much eye shadow, you can tell! The eye shadow might not be blended in, and it might be all over her face. It might be near her eyebrows and under her lower eyelids. This does not look good on anyone! You must be proportionate with your eye shadow wear. Apply eye shadow to only your eyelids below the crease, and you will avoid this problem. When you apply shadow to below the crease, it also prevents your shadow from smearing upwards and fading off. Many, many young girls wear excessive eye shadowing not knowing how to properly apply it. Less is more, ladies!

5) The number one mistake: Applying eyeliner wrong. The biggest mistake I see young girls make is the improper use of eyeliner. They fail to

realize that eyeliner is meant to be thin! It is not supposed to be a thick line. Wearing thick eyeliner is only going to make you look sleepy; also making your eyes appear very small and dull looking. You want your eyeliner to be super thin so that it opens up your eyes! You want to apply eyeliner to the lower lid, in a thin line, all the way under your eye. It goes under the entire eye, so don't leave out the corners of the eyes (inside and out). This is very important in applying eyeliner. Your eyes won't be defined to their maximum potential if applied improperly.

I really hope this book has helped introduce you to the basics of makeup and excited you for its real-world use. I hope that my directions were clear enough for you to properly apply your makeup when you go out and buy it. I have covered lots of material in this starter's book, including a tint of skin care, which is a very important process in the makeup world. Your skin must always be clean before you apply makeup, and always clean after you take it off. I gave you many of my personal tips of how to apply a variety of makeup components, which I hope you will incorporate and remember. I also wish you good luck when buying your first makeup products and finding your perfect shades. Thank you for purchasing my book, and I am looking forward to reading your feedback. Don't be afraid to try new things, go out there and experiment with all different colors, brands, and kinds of makeup. Good luck, young ladies!

Made in the USA
Middletown, DE
17 December 2020